Pocket Handbook of Body Reflex Zones Illustrated in Color

D1613258

by the same author

**Pocket Handbook of Particularly Effective Acupoints
for Common Conditions Illustrated in Color**
Guo Changqing Guoyan and Zhaiwei Liu Naigang
ISBN 978 1 84819 120 4
eISBN 978 0 85701 094 0

Pocket Handbook of Body Reflex Zones Illustrated in Color

Guo Changqing Guoyan
Zhaiwei Liu Naigang

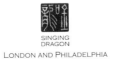

SINGING
DRAGON
LONDON AND PHILADELPHIA

Contributors: Cherui Taolin, Liangchuxi Duanlianhua, Zhongdingwen Zhanghuifang, Wuyuling Feifei, Renqiulan Liuqing, Liyuan Huangjuan, Yanghuijie Luyin

Additional translation work by Lucy Dean

First published in 2010 by People's Military Medical Press

This edition published in 2013
by Singing Dragon
an imprint of Jessica Kingsley Publishers
116 Pentonville Road
London N1 9JB, UK
and
400 Market Street, Suite 400
Philadelphia, PA 19106, USA

www.singingdragon.com

Library of Congress Cataloging in Publication Data
A CIP catalog record for this book is available from the Library of Congress

British Library Cataloguing in Publication Data
A CIP catalogue record for this book is available from the British Library

ISBN 978 1 84819 119 8
eISBN 978 0 85701 095 7

Printed and bound in China

CONTENTS

5. Reflex Zones of the Foot   109

About the Book

This book was compiled by professors of the School of Acupuncture, Moxibustion and Massage at Beijing University of Traditional Chinese Medicine, with the aim of creating a reflex zone therapy reference tool of both high academic and clinical relevance.

The book focuses on the reflex zones of the head, face, ears, hands and feet, introducing the location and indications of reflex zone therapy and the reflex zones themselves. The illustrated features offer a concise and practical way for readers to learn and remember basic applications.

The book provides a suitable pocket reference book for use in a clinical setting, as a teaching aid for teaching staff and students of Chinese medicine and for personal use for those with a special interest in reflex zone therapy.

The theory of reflex zone therapy is based on a holistic view of the body; an energy medicine understood through meridian and reflex theory. By applying certain stimuli to the reflex zones of the body, the healing of corresponding areas and pathologies can be instigated through the body's own adaptive regulation.

Reflex zone therapy has a long anecdotal history in China, but written records are sparse leaving no significant systematic theory. An early 20th century pioneer of modern reflexology, Dr. William Fitzgerald, inspired by Chinese acupuncture meridian theory, published a manual of regional therapies. Aside from this, medical workers in China, building on well-established Chinese medical theory, have developed, enriched and improved the use and understanding of the reflex zones of the head, face, ears and other areas commonly used in reflex zone therapy.

Reflex zone therapy aims to improve blood circulation, promote metabolism, achieve endocrine regulation, enhance immunity, and regulate and balance the role of the organs and their functions. Through careful diagnosis reflex zone therapy can be used in primary health care to achieve sustained and significant results. As a health care modality, reflex zone therapy is not only safe and effective, it is also simple to administer, economical, and practical, both in a health care setting and at home.

In order to promote the popularization and easy use of reflex zone therapy, this book introduces the more commonly used and most effective aspects of the theory, the zones of the head, face, ears, hands and feet. In this book the reader can find the locations and indications for reflex zone therapy and the specific reflex zones. The illustrated features offer a concise and practical way for readers to learn and remember basic applications.

CHAPTER 1

Cranial Reflex Zones

Cranial reflex zone therapy is a method by which acupuncture is applied to specific areas of the scalp to treat specific diseases. This practice is also known as scalp acupuncture and scalp penetration acupuncture therapy. The treatment lines that make up the reflex zones of scalp acupuncture therapy constitute a fundamental aspect of Chinese medical theory, and adhere to the principle of locating the points according to region, delineating the treatment line from the point in alignment with the channels. Accordingly there are 4 regions and 14 lines.

Midline of the Forehead

Location: On the midline of the forehead crossing the hairline by 0.5 cun, running 1 cun vertically downward from the point GV 24 shén ting Spirit Court.

Indications: Mental conditions and diseases of the head, nose, tongue, eyes and throat.

First Lateral Line of the Forehead

Location: On the forehead, lateral to the midline of the forehead directly above the medial corner of the eye (inner canthus of the eye). Crossing the hairline by 0.5 cun, running 1 cun vertically downward from the point BL 2 méi chōng Eyebrow Ascension.

Indications: Upper heater conditions of the lung and heart.

Second Lateral Line of the Forehead

Location: On the forehead, lateral to the 1st lateral line of the forehead directly above the pupil when looking straight ahead. Crossing the hairline by 0.5 cun, running 1 cun vertically downward from the point GB 15 tóu lín qì Head Supervising Tears.

Indications: Middle heater conditions of the spleen, stomach, liver and gallbladder.

Third Lateral Line of the Forehead

Location: On the forehead, lateral to the 2nd lateral line of the forehead directly above the lateral corner of the eye, 0.75 cun medial to the point ST 8 tóu wéi Head Binding (midway between the points GB 13 běn shén Original Spirit and ST 8 tóu wéi Head Binding). Crossing the hairline by 0.5 cun, running 1 cun vertically downward.

Indications: Lower heater conditions of the kidney and bladder.

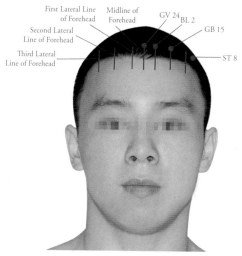

First Lateral Line of Forehead
Midline of Forehead
GV 24
BL 2
GB 15
Second Lateral Line of Forehead
Third Lateral Line of Forehead
ST 8

FIGURE 1.1

Central Vertex Line

Location: On the vertex of the head, on the central line of the scalp running in a posterior and anterior direction from the point GV 20 băi huì Hundred Meetings (on the midline of the scalp, 5 cun superior to the anterior hairline) to the point GV 21 qián dǐng Anterior Vertex (on the midline of the scalp, 3.5 cun superior to the anterior hairline).

Indications: Conditions of the lower back, legs and feet.

First Lateral Line of the Vertex

Location: On the vertex of the head, lateral to the central vertex line by 1.5 cun, running in a posterior direction for 1.5 cun from the point BL 7 tōngtiān Celestial Connection (on the scalp, 4 cun superior to the anterior hairline, 1.5 cun lateral to the midline of the head).

Indications: Conditions of the lower back, legs and feet; paralysis, numbness and pain in the lower extremities. In clinic this line is often used along with the central vertex line and upper ⅕ part of the anterior oblique line of the temporal vertex.

Second Lateral Line of the Vertex

Location: On the vertex of the head, lateral to the 1st lateral line of the vertex by 0.75 cun, running in a posterior direction for 1.5 cun from the point GB 17 zhèng yíng Upright Construction (on the scalp, 2.5 cun superior to the anterior hairline, directly superior to the pupil).

Indications: Conditions of the shoulders, arms and hands.

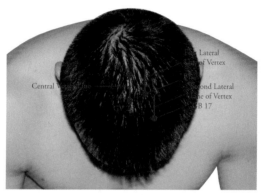

FIGURE 1.2

Anterior Oblique Line of the Temporal Vertex

Location: On the lateral aspect of the head, the line travels from the vertex to the temple from the anterior point of Ex-HN-1 qiánshéncōng

Anterior Spiritual Intelligence to GB 6 xuán lí Suspended Tuft.

Indications: Motor function disorders such as paralysis. The line can be divided into five parts; the upper ⅕ treating paralysis of the lower extremities, the central ⅖ treating paralysis of the upper extremities and the lower ⅖ treating facial paralysis, exercise induced aphasia and involuntary salivation.

Posterior Oblique Line of the Temporal Vertex

Location: On the lateral aspect of the head, the line travels from the vertex to the temple 1.5 cun posterior to the anterior oblique line of the temporal vertex, from the point GV 20 bǎi huì Hundred Meetings to the point GB 7 qū bìn Crook of the Temple.

Indications: Sensory function disorders such as pain, numbness and itching. The line can be divided into five parts; the upper ⅕ treating sensory abnormalities of the lower extremities, the central ⅖ treating sensory abnormalities of the upper extremities and the lower ⅔ treating sensory abnormalities of the head and face.

Anterior Temporal Line

Location: On the temporal aspect of the head within the temporal hairline, the line travels from the point GB 4 hàn yàn Forehead Fullness to GB 6 xuán lí Suspended Tuft.

Indications: Migraine, exercise induced aphasia, peripheral facial paralysis and oral diseases.

Posterior Temporal Line

Location: On the temporal aspect of the head, the line travels from the point GB 8 shuài gǔ Leading Valley to the point GB 7 qū bìn Crook of the Temple.

Indications: Migraine, vertigo, tinnitus and deafness.

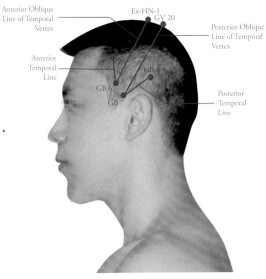

Anterior Oblique
Line of Temporal
Vertex

Ex-HN-1
GV 20

Posterior Oblique
Line of Temporal
Vertex

GB 6

Anterior
Temporal
Line

GB 8

GB 6

Posterior
Temporal
Line

GB 7

FIGURE 1.3

Upper Midline of the Occiput

Location: On the occiput, the line travels vertically over the center of the tuberosity of the occiput form from the point GV 18 qiáng jiān Strong Interval to GV 17 nǎo hù Brain Window.

Indications: Conditions of the eyes and pain in the lumbar vertebra.

Upper Lateral Line of the Occiput

Location: On the occiput, parallel to the midline of the occiput by a distance of 0.5 cun.

Indications: Conditions of the eyes and pain in the lumbar vertebra.

Lower Lateral Line of the Occiput

Location: On the occiput, below the tuberosity of the occiput, the vertical lines 2 cun in length travel from the point BL 9 yù zhěn Jade Pillow to the point BL 10 tiān zhù Celestial Pillar.

Indications: Conditions of the eyes and pain in the lumbar vertebra.

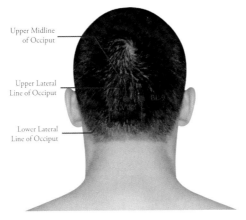

Upper Midline
of Occiput

Upper Lateral
Line of Occiput

Lower Lateral
Line of Occiput

FIGURE 1.4

CHAPTER 2

Facial Reflex Zones

Facial reflex zone therapy is a method of stimulating certain areas of the face in order to alleviate numerous conditions. The theory was developed upon the practice of diagnosis through the analysis of the complexion. The facial zones of the forehead, nose and upper lip can be divided into 7 reflex zones and the nose, eyes, mouth, cheeks and cheek bones constitute 17 further reflex zones.

Face

Location: The zone is situated in the exact center of the forehead.

Indications: Headache and dizziness.

Lung

Location: The point (M-HN-3 yìntáng Seal Temple) is situated at the midpoint of the line between the two medial ends of the eyebrows.

Indications: Cough and tightness in the chest.

Throat

Location: The point is situated at the midpoint of the line between the face zone and lung zone.

Indications: Inflammatory conditions of the throat (sore throat).

Heart

Location: The point (Root of the Mountain) is situated at the shallowest part of the bridge of the nose, at the center of the line between the two inner canthi of the eyes.

Indications: Palpitations and insomnia.

Lactation Point

Location: The point is situated midway between the heart point and the inner corner of the eye.

Indications: Limited lactation.

Liver

Location: The point is situated directly below the heart point, at the base of the bridge of the bone where it meets the nasal cartilage.

Indications: Pain in the side of the body and chest tightness.

Gallbladder

Location: The point is situated lateral to the liver point, directly below the inner corner of the eye, in the soft tissue below the nasal bone.

Indications: Nausea and vomiting.

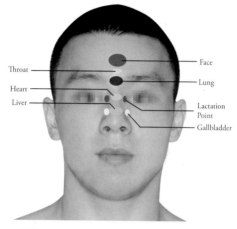

FIGURE 2.1

Spleen

Location: The point (Su Liao) is situated at the tip of the nose.

Indications: Malnourishment and poor appetite.

Bladder/Uterus

Location: The zone at the center of the filtrum at the point GV 26 rén zhōng Man's Center.

Indications: Dysmenorrhea.

Inner Thigh

Location: The zone is near ST 4 dì cāng Earth Granary, 0.5 cun lateral to the corner of the mouth at the meeting of the upper and lower lips.

Indications: Pain in the vastus medialis.

Stomach

Location: The zone is lateral to the spleen zone on the two sides of the nose.

Indications: Pain in the stomach.

Small Intestine

Location: The zone is situated at the center of the line between the gallbladder and the stomach zones.

Indications: Diarrhea.

Large Intestine

Location: The zone is situated directly below the outer canthus of the eye on the lower border of the cheek bone.

Indications: Constipation, abdominal pain and diarrhea.

Shoulder

Location: The zone is situated directly below the outer canthus of the eye lateral to the gallbladder point.

Indications: Shoulder and arm pain with an inability to flex.

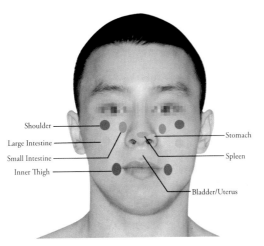

Shoulder

Large Intestine

Small Intestine

Inner Thigh

Stomach

Spleen

Bladder/Uterus

FIGURE 2.2

Arm

Location: At the intersection of the lines posterior to the shoulder zone and directly vertical to ST 7 xià guan Below the Bone.

Indications: Pain and inflammation of the shoulder and arm.

Hand

Location: Directly below the arm point, on the lower border of the zygomatic arch.

Indications: Pain and inflammation of the hand.

Back

Location: The point (SI 19 tīng gōng Auditory Palace) is situated 1 cun posterior to center of the cheek.

Indications: Lower back pain.

Kidney

Location: At the intersection of the line level with the inferior border of the nose and the line running vertically downward from the point Ex-HN-5 tài yang Supreme Yang.

Indications: Oliguria, dysuria and frequent urination.

Umbilicus

Location: 0.3 cun directly below the kidney point.

Indications: Abdominal pain.

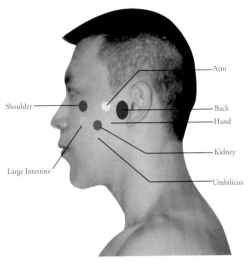

Shoulder

Arm

Back

Hand

Kidney

Umbilicus

Large Intestine

FIGURE 2.3

Thigh

Location: The zone is at the upper ⅓ of the line intersecting the earlobe and the mandibular angle.

Indications: Muscular sprain in the thigh.

Knee

Location: The zone is at the lower ⅓ of the line intersecting the earlobe and the mandibular angle.

Indications: Pain in the patella.

Patella

Location: The point (ST 6 jiá chē Jaw Bone) is situated in the depression superior to the mandibular angle.

Indications: Injury to the knee joint.

Shin

Location: Anterior to the mandibular angle, on the edge of the mandibular bone.

Indications: Ankle sprain and spasm of the gastrocnemius muscle.

Foot

Location: Anterior to the shin point, directly below the outer canthus of the eye, on the lower border of the mandible.

Indications: Ankle sprain and spasm of the gastrocnemius muscle.

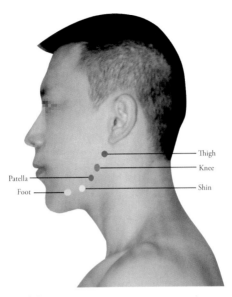

Thigh

Knee

Patella

Shin

Foot

FIGURE 2.4

CHAPTER 3

Auricular Reflex Zones

Auricular reflex zone therapy is a method of disease prevention and treatment through the stimulation of auricular points using either acupuncture needles or other forms of stimulation. In order to facilitate research and exchange, China was part of the working group by the World Health Organization Western Pacific Regional Office, to develop the auricular therapy international standardization program.

Section 1: Eight Points of the Ear Helix

Central Ear

Location: At the foot of the crus of the helix.

Indications: Hiccups, urticaria, pruritus, enuresis, hemoptysis.

Rectum

Location: Close to the notch of the crus of the helix, level with the colon point.

Indications: Constipation, diarrhea, rectal prolapse and hemorrhoids.

Urethra

Location: Superior to the rectum point on the crus of the helix, level with the bladder point.

Indications: Frequent and urgent urination, dysuria and urinary retention.

External Genitalia

Location: Superior to the urethra point on the crus of the helix, level with the sympathetic nervous system point.

Indications: Orchitis, epididymal inflammation and genital pruritus.

Anus

Location: On the helix, anterior to the foot of the antihelix of the ear.

Indications: Hemorrhoids and anal fissures.

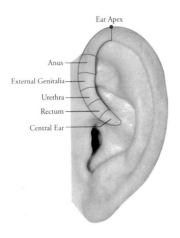

Figure 3.1

Ear Apex

Location: At the tip of the helix, opposite to the trailing edge at the foot of the antihelix.

Indications: Fever, high blood pressure and acute conjunctivitis.

Node

Location: On the auricular helix tubercle.

Indications: Dizziness, headache and high blood pressure.

Helix 1, Helix 2, Helix 3, Helix 4

Location: On the helix of the ear, whereby the helix is divided into four sections from the superior helix tubercle to the inferior helix notch, numbered Helix 1 to 4 consecutively.

Indications: Tonsillitis, upper respiratory tract infection, fever.

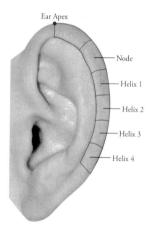

Ear Apex

Node

Helix 1

Helix 2

Helix 3

Helix 4

FIGURE 3.2

Section 2: Five Points of the Scapha and Antihelical Fold

Finger

Location: When the scapha and antihelical fold are divided into six parts starting at the superior depression and running vertically downward to the inferior helix notch, the finger zone constitutes the 1st part.

Indications: Paronychia (a skin infection occurring around the nails), finger pain and numbness.

Wind Stream

Location: When the scapha and antihelical fold are divided into six parts starting at the superior depression and running vertically downward to the inferior helix notch, wind stream is at the junction of the 1st and 2nd part; the finger and the wrist zones.

Indications: Urticaria, pruritus, allergic rhinitis.

Wrist

Location: When the scapha and antihelical fold are divided into six parts starting at the superior depression and running vertically downward to the inferior helix notch, the wrist constitutes the 2nd part.

Indications: Pain in the wrist area.

Elbow

Location: When the scapha and antihelical fold are divided into six parts starting at the superior depression and running vertically downward to the inferior helix notch, the elbow constitutes the 3rd part.

Indications: Humeral epicondylitis and pain in the elbow joint.

Shoulder

Location: When the scapha and antihelical fold are divided into six parts starting at the superior depression and running vertically downward to the inferior helix notch, the shoulder constitutes the 4th and 5th part.

Indications: Periarthritis and pain in the shoulder joint.

Clavicle

Location: When the scapha and antihelical fold are divided into six parts starting at the superior depression and running vertically downward to the inferior helix notch, the clavicle constitutes the 6th part.

Indications: Periarthritis of the shoulder joint.

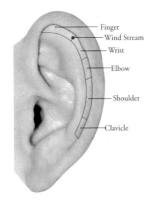

Finger
Wind Stream
Wrist
Elbow
Shoulder
Clavicle

FIGURE 3.3

Section 3: Five Points of the Superior Crura of the Antihelix

Toe

Location: The most superior and posterior part of the crura of the antihelix, adjacent to the apex of the ear.

Indications: Paronychia (a skin infection occurring around the nails), toe pain.

Heel

Location: The most superior and anterior part of the crura of the antihelix, adjacent to the upper part of the triangular fossa.

Indications: Pain in the heel.

Ankle

Location: Between the heel and the knee zones of the crura of the antihelix.

Indications: Ankle sprain.

Knee

Location: The central ⅓ of the crura of the antihelix.

Indications: Swelling and pain of the knee.

Hip

Location: The lower ⅓ of the crura of the antihelix.

Indications: Pain in the hip joint and sciatica.

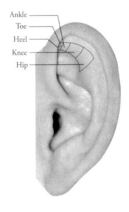

FIGURE 3.4

Section 4: Three Points of the Inferior Crura of the Antihelix

Buttock

Location: The posterior ⅓ of the inferior crura of the antihelix.

Indications: Hip fasciitis and sciatica.

Sciatic Nerve

Location: The anterior ⅔ of the inferior crura of the antihelix.

Indications: Sciatica.

Sympathetic Nervous System

Location: At the junction of the inferior crura of the helix and the foot of the helix.

Indications: Gastro-intestinal spasms, angina, biliary colic, ureteral calculi and functional neurological disorders.

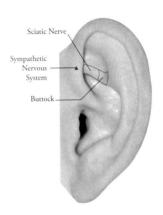

Sciatic Nerve

Sympathetic
Nervous
System

Buttock

FIGURE 3.5

Section 5: Six Points
of the Antihelix

Cervical Vertebra

Location: When the antihelix is vertically divided into five parts, the lower posterior part constitutes the cervical vertebra zone.

Indications: Stiff neck and cervical syndrome.

Thoracic Vertebra

Location: When the antihelix is vertically divided into five parts, the posterior central $\frac{2}{5}$ constitute the thoracic vertebra.

Indications: Thoracic and flank pain, premenstrual breast pain, mastitis insufficient lactation.

Lumbosacral Vertebra

Location: When the antihelix is vertically divided into five parts, the posterior upper $\frac{2}{5}$ constitute the lumbosacral vertebra.

Indications: Pain in the lumbosacral region.

Neck

Location: Anterior to the cervical vertebra zone, adjacent to the auricular cavum.

Indications: Stiffness, swelling and pain in the neck.

Chest

Location: Anterior to the thoracic vertebra zone, adjacent to the auricular cavum.

Indications: Thoracic and flank pain, congestion in the chest and mastitis.

Abdomen

Location: Anterior to the lumbosacral vertebra zone, adjacent to the auricular cavum.

Indications: Abdominal pain and distension, diarrhea and acute lumbar sprain.

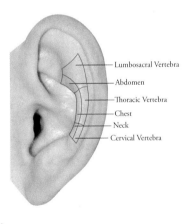

— Lumbosacral Vertebra
— Abdomen
— Thoracic Vertebra
— Chest
— Neck
— Cervical Vertebra

FIGURE 3.6

Section 6: Five Points of the Triangular Fossa

Spirit Door

Location: In the triangular fossa, when the distal ⅓ is bifurcated into two, spirit door constitutes the upper part.

Indications: Insomnia, copious dreaming, pain and withdrawal syndrome.

Pelvic Cavity

Location: In the triangular fossa, when the distal ⅓ is bifurcated into two, pelvic cavity constitutes the lower part.

Indications: Pelvic inflammatory disease.

Central Triangular Fossa

Location: When the triangular fossa is divided in three, central triangular fossa constitutes the central ⅓.

Indications: Asthma.

Internal Genitalia

Location: In the triangular fossa, when the medial ⅓ is bifurcated into two, internal genitalia lies in the depression in the lower part.

Indications: Dysmenorrhea, irregular menstruation, leucorrhea, dysfunction uterine bleeding, spermatorrhea and premature ejaculation.

Upper Triangular Fossa

Location: In the triangular fossa, when the medial ⅓ is bifurcated into two, upper triangular fossa lies in the superior medial part.

Indications: High blood pressure.

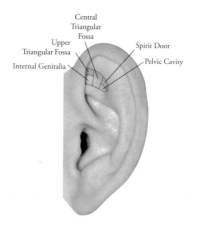

Central
Triangular
Fossa
Upper
Triangular Fossa
Internal Genitalia
Spirit Door
Pelvic Cavity

FIGURE 3.7

Section 7: Nine Points of the Tragus

Upper Tragus

Location: On the external surface of the tragus, in the area of the upper half.

Indications: Pharyngitis and simple obesity.

Lower Tragus

Location: On the external surface of the tragus, in the area of the lower half.

Indications: Rhinitis and simple obesity.

External Ear

Location: On the external surface of the tragus, superior to the upper tragus, at the junction of the tragus and the helix.

Indications: Otitis externa, otitis media and tinnitus.

External Nose

Location: At the center of the junction of the areas of the upper and lower tragus.

Indications: Inflammation of the nasal vestibule and rhinitis.

Apex of the Tragus

Location: On the external surface of the tragus, at the tip of the upper tragal notch.

Indications: Fever and tooth ache.

Adrenal Gland

Location: On the external surface of the tragus, at the tip of the lower tragal notch.

Indications: Low blood pressure, rheumatoid arthritis, mumps, malaria, drug induced vertigo.

Anterior Intertragal Notch

Location: On the external surface of the tragus, at the inferior most point of the external tragus at the base of the lower tragus.

Indications: Conditions of the eye.

Throat

Location: On the upper half of the internal surface of the tragus.

Indications: Hoarseness, sore throat and tonsillitis.

Internal Nose

Location: On the lower half of the internal surface of the tragus.

Indications: Rhinitis, sinusitis and epistaxis.

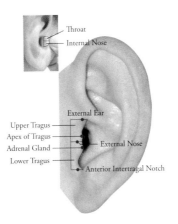

Throat
Internal Nose

External Ear
Upper Tragus
Apex of Tragus
Adrenal Gland — External Nose
Lower Tragus
Anterior Intertragal Notch

Figure 3.8

Section 8: Eight Points of the Antitragus

Apex of the Antitragus

Location: At the apex of the antitragus.

Indications: Asthma, mumps, pruritus, orchitis, epididymal inflammation.

Central Rim

Location: Midway between the apex of the antitragus and the junction of the antihelix and the antitragus.

Indications: Enuresis and inner ear vertigo.

Occiput

Location: The posterior superior portion of the antitragus.

Indications: Headache, dizziness, cough, epilepsy and neurasthenia.

Temple

Location: The central portion of the external surface of the antitragus.

Indications: Migraine.

Forehead

Location: The anterior inferior portion of the external surface of the antitragus.

Indications: Headache, dizziness, insomnia and copious dreaming.

Posterior Intertragal Notch

Location: Posterior to the base of the tragus, the point appears on the lower border of the antitragus.

Indications: Conditions of the eye.

Brainstem

Location: At the notch that marks the junction between the antihelix and the antitragus.

Indications: Headache, dizziness and pseudo-myopia.

Subcortex

Location: The interior surface of the antitragus.

Indications: Pain syndromes, malaria, neurasthenia and pseudo-myopia.

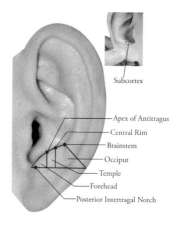

Subcortex

Apex of Antitragus
Central Rim
Brainstem
Occiput
Temple
Forehead
Posterior Intertragal Notch

FIGURE 3.9

Section 9: Eight Points Surrounding the Crus of the Helix

Colon

Location: The upper part of the superior portion surrounding the crus of the helix.

Indications: Diarrhea, constipation, dysentery, cough and acne.

Small Intestine

Location: The central part of the superior portion surrounding the crus of the helix.

Indications: Digestive disorders, abdominal pain, tachycardia, arrhythmia.

Appendix

Location: The point lies at the junction of the colon and small intestine zones.

Indications: Primary appendicitis and diarrhea.

Duodenum

Location: The lower part of the superior portion surrounding the crus of the helix.

Indications: Duodenal ulcer, cholecystitis, cholelithiasis, pylorospasm.

Stomach

Location: The area surrounding the terminal end of the crus of the helix.

Indications: Stomach cramps, gastritis, stomach ulcers, insomnia, tooth ache, indigestion.

Cardiac Region

Location: The posterior ⅓ of the area inferior to the crus of the helix.

Indications: Cardiac spasms, nervous vomiting.

Esophagus

Location: The central ⅓ of the area inferior to the crus of the helix.

Indications: Esophagitis, esophageal spasm, globus hystericus (difficulty swallowing).

Mouth

Location: The anterior ⅓ of the area inferior to the crus of the helix.

Indications: Facial paralysis, stomatitis, cholecystitis, cholelithiasis, withdrawal syndrome.

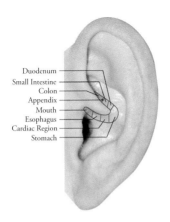

Duodenum
Small Intestine
Colon
Appendix
Mouth
Esophagus
Cardiac Region
Stomach

FIGURE 3.10

Section 10: Six Points of the Concha Cavity

Heart

Location: At the central point of the concha cavity.

Indications: Tachycardia, arrhythmia, angina, pulseless disease (Takayasu's disease), neurasthenia, hysteria, mouth sores.

Lung

Location: The portion of the concha cavity that surrounds the central point.

Indications: Cough, chest tightness, hoarseness, acne, skin pruritus, urticarial, measles, flat warts, constipation, withdrawal syndrome.

Trachea

Location: In the concha cavity, in the band running from the opening of the ear canal to the heart point.

Indications: Cough.

Spleen

Location: The posterior superior portion of the concha cavity.

Indications: Adnominal distension, diarrhea, constipation, anorexia, dysfunctional uterine bleeding, leukorrhagia, inner ear vertigo.

Endocrine System

Location: In the inferior portion of the concha cavity adjacent to the intertragic notch.

Indications: Dysmenorrhea, irregular menstruation, menopause syndrome, acne and malaria.

Three Heater

Location: In the inferior portion of the concha cavity, above the endocrine system zone.

Indications: Constipation, abdominal distension and pain in the upper limbs.

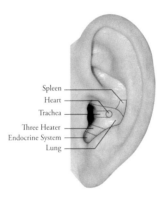

Spleen
Heart
Trachea
Three Heater
Endocrine System
Lung

FIGURE 3.11

Section 11: Seven Points of the Concha

Liver

Location: In the most posterior inferior segment of the concha.

Indications: Hypochondriac pain, dizziness, premenstrual stress disorder, irregular menstruation, menopausal syndrome, hypertension, pseudo-myopia, primary glaucoma.

Pancreas and Gallbladder

Location: In the concha, between the zones of the liver and the kidney.

Indications: Cholecystitis, cholelithiasis, bile duct ascariasis, migraine, herpes zoster, otitis media, tinnitus, hearing loss, acute pancreatitis.

Kidney

Location: In the concha, below the bifurcation of the antihelix.

Indications: Low back pain, tinnitus, neurasthenia, pyelonephritis, asthma, enuresis, irregular menstruation, nocturnal emission, premature ejaculation.

Bladder

Location: In the concha, anterior and inferior to the foot of the antihelix.

Indications: Cystitis, enuresis, urinary retention, low back pain, sciatica, occipital headache.

Ureter

Location: In the concha, between the two zones of the kidney and bladder.

Indications: Colic due to ureteral stones.

Corner of the Concha

Location: At the anterior superior corner of the concha.

Indications: Prostatitis, urethritis.

Center of the Superior Concha

Location: At the central point of the superior concha.

Indications: Abdominal pain, abdominal distension, ascariasis, mumps.

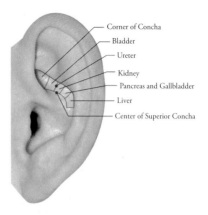

Corner of Concha
Bladder
Ureter
Kidney
Pancreas and Gallbladder
Liver
Center of Superior Concha

FIGURE 3.12

Section 12: Eight Points of the Auricular Lobule

The surface of the auricular lobule can be divided by three horizontal lines between the cartilage of the base of the tragus and the inferior edge of the lobule. Above the 2nd horizontal line, the area can be further divided by two vertical lines creating equal anterior and posterior portions.

The result is to divide the lobule into nine equal parts.

Teeth
Location: Part 1 (see Figure 3.13).
Indications: Tooth ache, periodontitis and low blood pressure.

Tongue
Location: Part 2 (see Figure 3.13).
Indications: Glossitis, stomatitis.

Jaw
Location: Part 3 (see Figure 3.13).
Indications: Tooth ache, temporomandibular joint dysfunction.

Anterior Ear Lobe
Location: Part 4 (see Figure 3.13).
Indications: Tooth ache, neurasthenia.

Eye

Location: Part 5 (see Figure 3.13).

Indications: Acute conjunctivitis, electric ophthalmia, blepharitis, pseudomyopia.

Inner Ear

Location: Part 6 (see Figure 3.13).

Indications: Inner ear vertigo, tinnitus, reduced hearing.

Cheek

Location: At the center of the junction of the 5th and 6th parts (see Figure 3.13).

Indications: Peripheral facial paralysis, trigeminal neuralgia, acne and flat warts.

Tonsils

Location: Parts 7, 8, and 9 (see Figure 3.13).

Indications: Tonsillitis and pharyngitis.

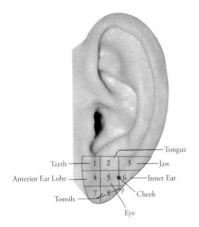

Teeth — 1 2 3 — Jaw
Tongue
Anterior Ear Lobe — 4 5 6 — Inner Ear
Cheek
Tonsils — 7 8 9
Eye

FIGURE 3.13

Section 13: Nine Points of the Posterior Ear

Upper Ear Root

Location: The most superior aspect of the posterior ear root.

Indications: Epistaxis.

Root of the Ear Vagus

Location: At the root of the ear where the posterior root meets the mastoid process, on the posterior aspect of the helix foot.

Indications: Cholecystitis, cholelithiasis, bile duct ascariasis, nasal congestion, tachycardia, abdominal pain, diarrhea.

Lower Ear Root

Location: The most inferior aspect of the posterior ear root.

Indications: Low blood pressure.

Posterior Ear Groove

Location: The concave groove runs in a "Y" shape from the upper and lower crus of the antihelix along the backbone of the helix.

Indications: High blood pressure, pruritus.

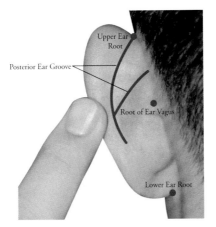

FIGURE 3.14

Heart Point on the Posterior Surface

Location: The upper ⅓ of the posterior ear.

Indications: Palpitations, insomnia and copious dreams.

Spleen Point on the Posterior Surface

Location: The lateral ⅓ of the central part of the posterior ear.

Indications: Stomach ache, indigestion and lack of appetite.

Liver Point on the Posterior Surface

Location: The central ⅓ of the central part of the posterior ear.

Indications: Cholecystitis, cholelithiasis, hypochondriac pain.

Lung Point on the Posterior Surface

Location: The inferior ⅓ of the posterior ear, directly below the spleen point of the posterior ear.

Indications: Cough, skin pruritus.

Kidney Point on the Posterior Surface

Location: The medial ⅓ of the central part of the posterior ear.

Indications: Headache, dizziness and neurasthenia.

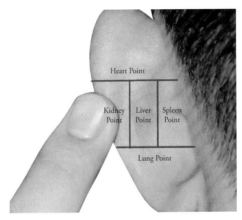

FIGURE 3.15

CHAPTER 4

Reflex Zones of the Hand

Reflex zone therapy of the hands is a method of stimulating zones on the hands in order to treat certain conditions of the body. As early as the text the *Yellow Emperor's Internal Classic* there was extensive discussion of the diagnostic properties of the hands along with the occurrence of numerous antique points appearing on the hands. In the 1970s, Chinese medical practitioners further perfected the use of reflex zone therapy of the hand through analysis of meridian theory and clinical practice.

Frontal Sinus

Location: At the tips of the five fingers.

Indications: Stroke, concussion, sinusitis, dizziness, headache, colds, fever, insomnia and conditions of the eyes, ears, mouth and nose.

Brain (Head)

Location: The palmar aspect of the head of the thumb.

Indications: Concussion, stroke, cerebral palsy, cerebral thrombosis, dizziness, headache, cold, delirium, neurasthenia and visual impairment.

Pituitary Gland

Location: The central point of the palmar aspect of the head of the thumb.

Indications: Dysfunctional conditions of the thyroid, parathyroid, adrenal gland, gonads, spleen and pancreas, menopausal syndrome, stunted growth in children.

Nose

Location: On the lateral aspect of the head of the thumb, where the skin changes texture.

Indications: Nasal congestion, runny nose, epistaxis (nose bleed), sinusitis, allergic rhinitis, acute and chronic rhinitis and upper respiratory tract infections.

Tonsils

Location: On the proximal phalanx of the thumb, either side of the proximal dorsal tendon.

Indications: Tonsillitis, upper respiratory tract infection and fever.

A. Frontal Sinus

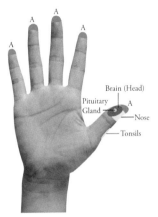

FIGURE 4.1

Esophagus and Trachea

Location: On the radial side of the proximal phalanx of the thumb, where the skin changes texture.

Indications: Esophagitis, esophageal cancer and bronchitis.

Respiratory Organs of the Chest

Location: On the lateral aspect of the thenar eminence, running between the transverse crease of the wrist and the transverse crease of the metacarpophalangeal joint.

Indications: Chest tightness, wheezing, cough, pneumonia, bronchitis and asthma.

Stomach

Location: The distal part of the 1st metacarpal bone.

Indications: Stomach pain, distension, excessive stomach acid, indigestion, ptosis of the stomach, nausea, vomiting, acute and chronic gastritis.

Pancreas

Location: Between the reflex zones of the stomach and the duodenum, at the central portion of the 1st metacarpal bone.

Indications: Pancreatitis, diabetes and indigestion.

Duodenum

Location: On the palmar aspect of the hand, at the proximal portion of the 1st metacarpal bone, inferior to the reflex zone of the pancreas.

Indications: Duodenal ulcers, a lack of appetite, indigestion, abdominal distension and food poisoning.

Thyroid

Location: On the palmar aspect of the hand, between the 1st and 2nd metacarpal bones, following the curved line of the thenar from the transverse crease of the wrist to the margin of the web.

Indications: Both hyperthyroidism and hypothyroidism, thyroiditis, heart palpitations, insomnia, common cold, irritability and obesity.

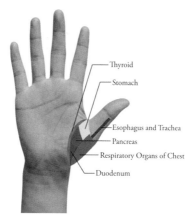

Figure 4.2

Eyes

Location: On both the palmar and dorsal aspects of the proximal phalanx of the 1st and 2nd fingers.

Indications: Conjunctivitis, keratitis, myopia, hyperopia, glaucoma, cataracts, photophobia, tearing, presbyopia and retinal hemorrhage.

Ears

Location: On both the palmar and dorsal aspects of the proximal phalanx of the 3rd and 4th fingers.

Indications: Tinnitus, ear infections and hearing loss.

Trapezius

Location: On the palmar side of the hand, in the strip between the eye and ear reflex zones.

Indications: Neck, shoulder and back pain, cervical spondylosis, stiff neck.

Anterior Neck and Shoulder

Location: In the web at the base of the fingers between the proximal phalanxes and the metacarpophalangeal joints; the dorsal aspect is used for treating the posterior shoulder and neck conditions, whereas the palmar aspect is used to treat anterior shoulder and neck conditions.

Indications: Neck and shoulder pain, frozen shoulder, cervical spondylosis, neck and shoulder fasciitis and a stiff neck.

Neck

Location: The medial aspect of the proximal phalanx of the thumb, both on the palmar and dorsal aspects.

Indications: Neck pain, stiff neck, dizziness, headache, nosebleed, high blood pressure and stiff neck.

A. Anterior Neck and Shoulder
B. Ears
C. Eyes

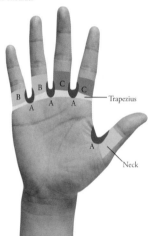

FIGURE 4.3

Bladder

Location: In the depression between the thenar eminence and the hypothenar eminence.

Indications: Cystitis, urethritis, bladder stones, high blood pressure, atherosclerosis, urinary tract and bladder disorders.

Ureter

Location: On the palm, in the strip between the bladder reflex zone and the kidney reflex zone.

Indications: Ureteritis, ureteral stones, ureteral stenosis, hypertension, arteriosclerosis, rheumatism, urinary tract infections.

Kidney

Location: In the palm, at the midpoint of the 3rd metacarpal bone, at the location of PC 8 láo gong Palace of Labor.

Indications: Nephritis, kidney stones, a wandering kidney, renal dysfunction, uremia, lower back pain, urinary tract infection, hypertension and edema.

Adrenal Glands

Location: On the palm, between the heads of the 2nd and 3rd carpal bones.

Indications: Dizziness, hypertension, fingertip paralysis, sweating palms, adrenocortical insufficiency.

Celiac Plexus

Location: On the palm, between the heads of the 2nd and 3rd carpal bones and between the heads of the 3rd and the 4th carpal bones, either side of the kidney reflex zone.

Indications: Gastro-intestinal disorders, abdominal pain, abdominal distension, diarrhea, hiccups, menopausal syndrome, irritability and insomnia.

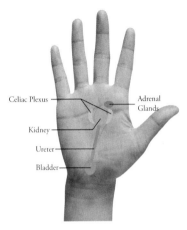

Celiac Plexus

Adrenal Glands

Kidney

Ureter

Bladder

FIGURE 4.4

Ascending Colon

Location: On the palmar aspect of the right hand, in the area from between the 4th and 5th metacarpal bones to the thenar eminence.

Indications: Constipation, abdominal pain, enteritis and diarrhea.

Transverse Colon

Location: On the palmar aspect of the right hand, in a band superior to the reflex zone of the ascending colon; the right hand, in the area from between the 4th and 5th metacarpal bones to the thenar eminence.

Indications: Diarrhea, abdominal distension, abdominal pain, colitis and constipation.

Cecum and Appendix

Location: On the palmar aspect of the right hand, where the base of the 4th and 5th metacarpal bones meet the hamate bone near the ulnar.

Indications: Abdominal distension, diarrhea, indigestion and appendicitis.

Ileocecal Valve

Location: On the palmar aspect of the right hand, where the base of the 4th and 5th metacarpal bones meet the hamate bone on the radial side.

Indications: Abdominal distension and pain.

Small Intestine

Location: On the concave center of the palmar aspect of both hands, surrounded by the reflex zones of intestines.

Indications: Acute and chronic enteritis, indigestion, a lack of appetite and nausea.

Stomach, Spleen and Colon

Location: On the palmar aspect of the hand, in an oval shape between the 1st and 2nd metacarpal bones.

Indications: Indigestion, a lack of appetite, abdominal pain and distension, diarrhea, gastritis and constipation.

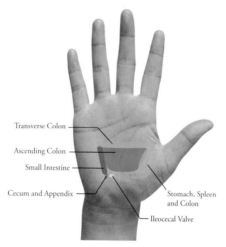

Transverse Colon

Ascending Colon

Small Intestine

Cecum and Appendix

Stomach, Spleen
and Colon

Ileocecal Valve

FIGURE 4.5

Lung and Bronchus

Location: The reflex zone of the lung is on the palmar aspect of the hand, running along the heads of the 2nd, 3rd, 4th, and 5th metacarpal bones in a band along the metacarpophalangeal joints. The reflex zone of the bronchus extends along the proximal phalange of the middle finger.

Indications: Pneumonia, bronchitis, emphysema, tuberculosis, lung cancer and congestion in the chest.

Liver

Location: On the palmar aspect of the right hand, between the heads of the 4th and 5th metacarpal bones.

Indications: Hepatitis, cirrhosis of the liver, abdominal pain, indigestion, abdominal distension, dizziness and conditions of the eye.

Gallbladder

Location: On the palmar aspect of the right hand, between the heads of the 4th and 5th metacarpal bones, in the area on the wrist side of the reflex zone of the liver.

Indications: Cholecystitis, cholelithiasis, bile duct ascariasis, anorexia, dyspepsia, gastrointestinal disorders, hyperlipidemia and acne.

Gonads (Testes and Ovaries)

Location: At the root of both palms, in the center of the transverse carpal ligament, in the equivalent position as PC 7 dà líng Great Mount.

Indications: Sexual dysfunction, infertility, benign prostatic hyperplasia, menstrual irregularity and dysmenorrhea.

Prostate, Uterus, Vagina and Urethra

Location: At the root of both palms, along the transverse carpal ligament, running either side of the reflex zone of the gonads.

Indications: Prostatic hyperplasia, prostatitis, uterine fibroids, endometritis, cervicitis, vaginitis, abnormal vaginal discharge, urethritis and urinary tract infections.

Groin

Location: At the root of both palms, on the transverse carpal ligament, in the depression at the head of the radius. In the equivalent position as LU 7 tài yuān The Great Abyss.

Indications: Sexual dysfunction, benign prostatic hyperplasia, reproductive system disorders, hernia and abdominal pain.

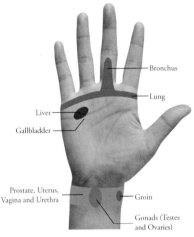

Bronchus
Lung
Liver
Gallbladder
Prostate, Uterus,
Vagina and Urethra
Groin
Gonads (Testes
and Ovaries)

FIGURE 4.6

Heart

Location: On the ulnar side of the left hand, on both the palmar and dorsal aspects of the hand between the distal ends of the 4th and 5th metacarpal bones.

Indications: Arrhythmia, angina, palpitations, chest tightness, high blood pressure, low blood pressure, heart defects and conditions of the circulatory system.

Spleen

Location: On the palmar aspect of the left hand, between the distal ends of the 4th and 5th metacarpal bones.

Indications: A lack of appetite, dyspepsia, fever, inflammation and anemia.

Descending Colon

Location: On the palmar aspect of the left hand, between the 4th and 5th metacarpal bones in a band between the head of the metacarpals and the hamate bone.

Indications: Diarrhea, abdominal pain, abdominal distension, colitis and constipation.

Sigmoid Colon

Location: On the palmar aspect of the left hand, in a band from the base of 5th metacarpal bone, where it meets the hamate bone, to where it meets the base of the 1st and 2nd metacarpal bones.

Indications: Abdominal pain and distension, diarrhea, colitis and constipation.

Anus and Anal Canal

Location: On the palmar aspect of the left hand, at the junction of the 2nd carpometacarpal joint, at the radial end of the reflex zone of the sigmoid colon.

Indications: Constipation, rectal prolapse and hemorrhoids.

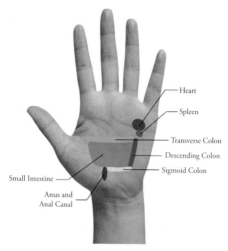

Heart
Spleen
Transverse Colon
Descending Colon
Sigmoid Colon
Small Intestine
Anus and
Anal Canal

FIGURE 4.7

Cerebellum and Brainstem

Location: On the palmar surface of the head of the thumb, on the ulna aspect.

Indications: Concussion, hypertension, dizziness, headache, insomnia, colds, difficulty walking, muscle tension, tendon and joint conditions.

Trigeminal Nerve

Location: On the distal, palmar surface of the head of the thumb, on the ulna aspect, distal to the reflex zone of the cerebellum and brainstem.

Indications: Facial nerve paralysis, migraine, neuralgia, insomnia, common cold, mumps and nerve pain in the eyes, ears and mouth.

Upper and Lower Jaw

Location: On the dorsal aspect of the thumb, in a band over the crease of the interphalangeal joint. Above the crease is used in the treatment of conditions of the upper jaw and below the crease is used for lower jaw conditions.

Indications: Temporomandibular joint disorders, periodontitis, gingivitis, dental caries and oral ulcers.

Tongue

Location: On the dorsal aspect of the thumb, at the central point of the crease of the interphalangeal joint.

Indications: Mouth ulcers and dysgeusia.

Larynx and Trachea

Location: At the midpoint of the dorsal aspect of the metacarpal bone of the thumb.

Indications: Upper respiratory tract infection, pharyngitis, bronchitis, cough and asthma.

Tonsils

Location: On the dorsal aspect of the metacarpal bone of the thumb, either side of the tendon.

Indications: Tonsillitis, upper respiratory tract infection and fever.

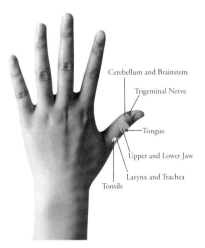

Cerebellum and Brainstem

Trigeminal Nerve

Tongue

Upper and Lower Jaw

Larynx and Trachea

Tonsils

FIGURE 4.8

Spine

Location: On the dorsal aspect of the hand between the 1st, 2nd, 3rd, 4th and 5th metacarpal bones, including the reflex zones of cervical spine, the thoracic spine, the lumbar spine, the sacrum and the coccyx.

Indications: Conditions of the cervical vertebra, stiff neck, back ache and lower back pain.

Cervical Spine

Location: On the dorsal aspect of the hand, the distal ⅓ of the space between the metacarpal bones.

Indications: Neck stiffness, neck pain, dizziness, headache, stiff neck and cervical conditions.

Thoracic Spine

Location: On the dorsal aspect of the hand, the central ⅔ of the space between the metacarpal bones.

Indications: Shoulder pain, thoracic bone spurs, lumbar pain, thoracic disc conditions, chest tightness and pain in the chest.

Lumbar Spine

Location: On the dorsal aspect of the hand, the proximal ⅔ of the space between the metacarpal bones.

Indications: Back pain, lumbar spine bone spurs, lumbar pain, lumbar disc conditions, lumbar muscle strain.

Sacrum

Location: On the dorsal aspect of the hand, five points at the junction of the carpometacarpal joint.

Indications: Sacral injuries, sacral bone spurs and sciatica.

Coccyx

Location: On the dorsal aspect of the hand, on the posterior transverse crease of the wrist.

Indications: Sciatica, sequelae of coccyx injuries.

Ribs

Location: On the dorsum of the hand, the medial reflex point of the ribs is located on the radial side of the center of the 2nd metacarpal bone, the lateral reflex point of the ribs is located in the depression between the base of the 4th and 5th metacarpal bones.

Indications: Pleurisy, tightness of the chest, injury to the rib.

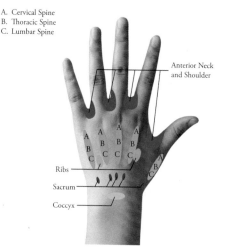

A. Cervical Spine
B. Thoracic Spine
C. Lumbar Spine

Anterior Neck
and Shoulder

Ribs

Sacrum

Coccyx

FIGURE 4.9

Labyrinthine

Location: On the dorsum of the hand, at the junction of the 3rd, 4th and 5th metacarpalphalangeal joints and the base of the 3rd, 4th and 5th fingers.

Indications: Dizziness, tinnitus, Meniere's syndrome, motion sickness, high blood pressure, low blood pressure and balance disorders.

Chest and Breast

Location: On the dorsum of the hand, in a band across the heads of the 2nd, 3rd and 4th metacarpal bones.

Indications: Chest conditions, respiratory diseases, heart disease and conditions of the breasts.

Diaphragm

Location: On the dorsum of the hand, in a band across the center of the 2nd, 3rd, 4th and 5th metacarpal bones.

Indications: Hiccups, nausea, vomiting, abdominal distension and abdominal pain.

Blood Pressure

Location: On the dorsum of the hand, the area enclosed by the 1st and 2nd metacarpal bones and LI 5 yáng xī Yang River, reaching half way up the radial side of the proximal phalanges of the index finger.

Indications: High and low blood pressure, dizziness and headache.

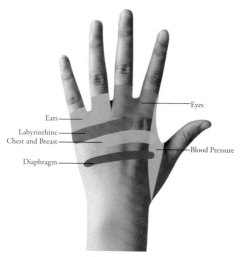

Ears
Labyrinthine
Chest and Breast
Diaphragm
Eyes
Blood Pressure

FIGURE 4.10

Shoulder Joint

Location: Distal to the metacarpophalangeal joint of the little finger, where the skin changes texture.

Indications: Frozen shoulder, arm pain, numbness in the hands and cataract.

Elbow Joint

Location: On the dorsal aspect of the hand, the central portion of the ulna side of the 5th metacarpal bone.

Indications: Conditions of the elbow diseases (such as tennis elbow, olecranon bursitis, medial epicondylosis), upper limb paralysis and arm numbness.

Knee Joint

Location: On the ulna edge of the proximal 5th metacarpal bone in the depression on the wrist.

Indications: Lesions (such as osteoarthritis of the knee, infrapatellar bursitis, meniscus injury, ligament injury) and paralysis of the lower limb.

Hip Joint

Location: On the dorsum of the hand, around the junction of the ulnar and the radial aspect of the styloid process.

Indications: Conditions of the hips, sciatica and lower back pain.

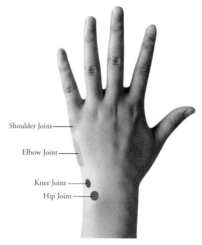

Shoulder Joint

Elbow Joint

Knee Joint

Hip Joint

FIGURE 4.11

Lymph Nodes of the Head and Neck

Location: On the dorsum of the hand, in the depression in the web between the fingers.

Indications: Swollen lymph nodes in the neck, goiter, hyperthyroidism and tooth ache.

Parathyroid

Location: On the dorsum of the hand, in the depression on the radial side of the 1st metacarpal bone, proximal to the head.

Indications: Allergies, cramps, insomnia, vomiting, nausea, low calcium levels, brittle nails, epileptic seizures.

Thymus Lymph Node

Location: On the dorsum of the hand, on the ulnar side of the first metacarpophalangeal joint.

Indications: Fever, inflammation, cysts, and used to enhance the immune system's ability to fight cancer.

Upper Body Lymph Nodes

Location: On the dorsum of the hand, at the junction of the lunate, triangular and ulna bones.

Indications: Fever, inflammation, cysts, and used to enhance the immune ability to fight cancer.

Lower Body Lymph Nodes

Location: On the dorsum of the hand, at the junction of the navicular and radius bones.

Indications: Fever, inflammation and cysts.

A. Lymph Nodes of the Head and Neck

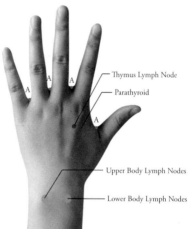

FIGURE 4.12

CHAPTER 5

Reflex Zones of the Foot

Reflex zone therapy of the feet is a method of stimulating zones on the feet in order to treat certain conditions of the body. The reflex zones of the foot cover the whole area of the foot leading to the lower leg. It is also known as maintenance of health through foot reflexology or reflexive band therapy.

Brain

Location: In the horizontal band on the pad of the distal phalanx of the big toe. For conditions of the left cerebellum treat the left toe and for conditions of the right cerebellum treat the right toe.

Indications: Concussion, stroke, cerebral palsy, cerebral thrombosis, dizziness, headache, cold, delirium, neurasthenia and visual impairment.

Frontal Sinus

Location: The tip of the five toes.

Indications: Stroke, concussion, sinusitis, dizziness, headache, common cold, fever, insomnia and conditions of the eyes, ears, mouth and nose.

Cerebellum and Brainstem

Location: On the medial aspect of the 1st proximal phalanx, near the root of the 2nd toe.

Indications: Concussion, hypertension, dizziness, headache, insomnia, common cold, difficulty walking, muscle tension, tendon and joint conditions.

Pituitary

Location: At the center point of the horizontal band on the pad of the distal phalanx of the big toe.

Indications: Thyroid, parathyroid, adrenal glands, gonads, spleen, pancreas, stunted growth in children and menopausal syndrome.

Trigeminal Nerve

Location: On the medial aspect of the 1st distal phalanx, near the junction with the 2nd toe (medial to the reflex zone of the brain).

Indications: Thyroid, parathyroid, adrenal glands, gonads, spleen, pancreas, stunted growth in children and menopausal syndrome.

Nose

Location: On the lateral aspect of the pad of the distal phalanx of the big toe, from near the tip of the toe to the base of the 1st distal phalanx.

Indications: Nasal congestion, runny nose, nasal bleeding (bleeding conditions), sinusitis, allergic rhinitis, acute and chronic rhinitis and upper respiratory tract infection.

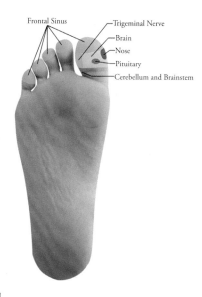

Frontal Sinus
Trigeminal Nerve
Brain
Nose
Pituitary
Cerebellum and Brainstem

FIGURE 5.1

Eye

Location: At the base of the 2nd and 3rd toes covering the 1st proximal phalanx and the metatarsophalangeal joint. For conditions of the left eye treat the left foot and for conditions of the right eye treat the right foot.

Indications: Conjunctivitis, keratitis, myopia, hyperopia, glaucoma, cataract, photophobia, lacrimation, presbyopia and retinal hemorrhage.

Ear

Location: At the base of the 4th and 5th toes covering the 1st proximal phalanx and the metatarsophalangeal joint. For conditions of the left ear treat the left foot and for conditions of the right eye treat the right foot.

Indications: Tinnitus, ear infections and hearing loss.

Trapezius

Location: At the base of 2nd, 3rd and 4th toes, in a ribbon along the metatarsophalangeal joint.

Indications: Frozen shoulder, shoulder pain, weakness in the arms and numbness of the hands, stiff neck and cataracts.

Neck

Location: In a band on the plantar aspect at the base of the 1st proximal phalanx.

Indications: Neck pain, stiff neck, dizziness, headaches, nosebleeds, high blood pressure, stiff neck.

Cervical Vertebra

Location: In a band running along the medial aspect of the 1st proximal phalanx.

Indications: Neck stiffness, neck pain, dizziness, headache, stiff neck and cervical lesions.

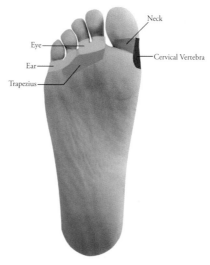

Neck

Eye

Ear

Trapezius

Cervical Vertebra

FIGURE 5.2

Lung and Bronchus

Location: In a band along the 2nd, 3rd, 4th and 5th metatarsophalangeal joint, with a protrusion in the center along the 3rd toe to the proximal phalanx.

Indications: Pneumonia, bronchitis, emphysema, tuberculosis, lung cancer and chest tightness.

Adrenal Gland

Location: On the plantar aspect of the foot, slightly lateral to the head of the 2nd metatarsal bone.

Indications: Inflammation, asthma, allergies, irregular heartbeat, fainting, rheumatism, arthritis and adrenal cortex imperfecta.

Thyroid

Location: On the plantar aspect of the foot in an "L" shaped band running between the heads of the 1st and 2nd metatarsal bones and between the body and the head of the 1st metatarsal bone.

Indications: Hyper and hypothyroidism, thyroiditis, heart palpitations, insomnia, common cold, irritability and obesity.

Parathyroid

Location: On the medial edge of the head of the 1st metatarsal bone, lateral to the ball of the foot.

Indications: Allergies, cramps, insomnia, vomiting, nausea, low calcium, brittle nails and epileptic seizures.

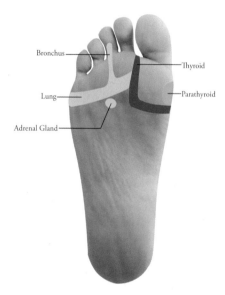

Bronchus

Lung

Adrenal Gland

Thyroid

Parathyroid

FIGURE 5.3

Esophagus

Location: In a thin strip on the plantar aspect of the field, covering the head of the 1st metatarsal bone.

Indications: Esophageal cancer and conditions of the esophagus.

Stomach

Location: On the sole of the foot in the center of the 1st metatarsal bone, just proximal to the head.

Indications: Stomach pain, bloating, excessive stomach acid, indigestion, ptosis of the stomach, nausea, vomiting, acute and chronic gastritis.

Pancreas

Location: On the sole of the foot, at the distal end of the 1st metatarsal bone, between the reflex zones of the stomach and the duodenum.

Indications: Pancreatitis, diabetes and indigestion.

Duodenum

Location: On the sole of the foot, at the proximal end of the 1st metatarsal bone, where it meets the cuneiform joint.

Indications: Duodenal ulcer, a lack of appetite, indigestion, intestinal distension, food retention.

Heart

Location: On the sole of the foot, between the distal heads of the 4th and 5th metatarsal bones.

Indications: Arrhythmia, angina, palpitations, chest tightness, hypertension, hypotension, heart defects and diseases of the circulatory system.

Spleen

Location: On the sole of the left foot, between the proximal ends of the 4th and 5th metatarsal bones.

Indications: A lack of appetite, dyspepsia, fever, inflammation and anemia.

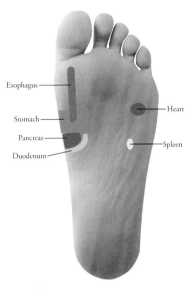

Esophagus

Heart

Stomach

Pancreas

Spleen

Duodenum

FIGURE 5.4

Liver

Location: On the sole of the right foot, between the distal ends of the 4th and 5th metatarsal bones.

Indications: Hepatitis, cirrhosis, hepatomegaly, dry mouth, eye problems, a loss of appetite, constipation and conditions of the gallbladder.

Gallbladder

Location: On the sole of the right foot, between the 4th and 5th metatarsal bones in the center.

Indications: Cholecystitis, gallstones, jaundice, conditions of the liver, a lack of appetite and constipation.

Celiac Plexus

Location: In the center of the sole of the foot, in an area covering the 2nd, 3rd and 4th metatarsal bones.

Indications: Back pain, chest tightness, hiccups, stomach cramps and bloating.

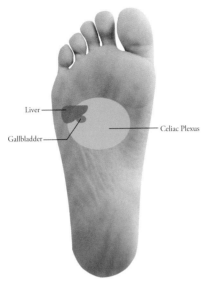

Liver

Gallbladder

Celiac Plexus

FIGURE 5.5

Transverse Colon

Location: On the sole of the foot, in a band traversing the proximal ends of the 1st to 5th metatarsal bones.

Indications: Diarrhea, bloating, abdominal pain, colitis and constipation.

Ascending Colon

Location: On the right foot, in a vertical band along the lateral edge of the reflex zone of the small intestine.

Indications: Constipation, abdominal pain, enteritis and diarrhea.

Small Intestine

Location: On the depression in the center of the sole of the foot, the square shape around the junction of the cuneiform, cuboid and navicular bones.

Indications: Acute and chronic enteritis, indigestion, a lack of appetite, nausea with stomach distension, dull pain in the abdomen, fatigue and tension.

Ileocecal Valve

Location: On the right sole of the foot, anterior to the calcaneus bone on the lateral edge, anterior to the reflex zone of the appendix.

Indications: Digestion and absorption disorders.

Cecum and Appendix

Location: On the sole of the right foot, anterior to the calcaneus bone on the lateral edge.

Indications: Appendicitis and abdominal distension.

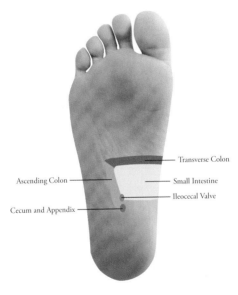

Transverse Colon

Ascending Colon — Small Intestine

— Ileocecal Valve

Cecum and Appendix —

FIGURE 5.6

Descending Colon

Location: On the sole of the left foot, in a band lateral to the cuboid bone.

Indications: Diarrhea, abdominal pain, bloating, colitis and constipation.

Rectum and Sigmoid

Location: On the sole of the left foot, in a horizontal band anterior to the calcaneus bone.

Indications: Abdominal pain, bloating, diarrhea, enteritis and constipation.

Anus

Location: On the sole of the left foot, anterior to the calcaneus bone at the medial end of the reflex zone of the rectum and sigmoid.

Indications: Constipation, rectal prolapse and hemorrhoids.

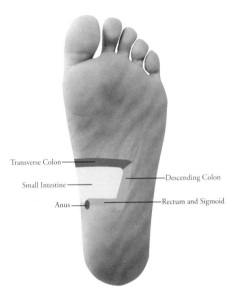

Transverse Colon

Small Intestine

Anus

Descending Colon

Rectum and Sigmoid

FIGURE 5.7

Kidney

Location: On the sole of the foot, between the junctions of the lower ends of the 2nd and 3rd metatarsal bones.

Indications: Nephritis, kidney stones, wandering kidney, renal dysfunction, uremia, lower back pain, urinary tract infections and high blood pressure.

Urethra

Location: On the sole of the foot, in an arch shaped band running from the reflex zone of the kidney to the reflex zone of the bladder.

Indications: Nephritis, kidney stones, wandering kidney, renal dysfunction, uremia, lower back pain, urinary tract infections and high blood pressure.

Bladder

Location: On the medial aspect of the sole of the foot, anterior to the medial malleolus and adjacent to the abductor muscle attachment on the inferior scaphoid bone.

Indications: Cystitis, urethritis, bladder stones, high blood pressure, atherosclerosis, urinary tract and bladder disorders.

Gonads (Testes and Ovaries)

Location: (1) In the center of the heel of the foot. (2) Below and distal to the lateral malleolus, in the triangular zone formed there.

Indications: Dysmenorrhea, irregular menstruation, infertility, sexual dysfunction, menopausal syndrome. Reflex zones in the heel are generally named the insomnia zone, and are particularly effective in treating insomnia.

Insomnia Point

Location: On the sole of the heel anterior to the calcaneus bone, distal to the reflex zone of the gonads.

Indications: Particularly effective in the treatment of insomnia. Insomnia, copious dreaming, headache and dizziness.

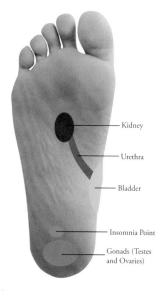

- Kidney
- Urethra
- Bladder
- Insomnia Point
- Gonads (Testes and Ovaries)

FIGURE 5.8

Prostate and Uterus

Location: On the medial aspect of the heel bone, in the triangular depression posterior and distal to the medial malleolus.

Indications: In male patients: prostatitis, prostatic hypertrophy, frequent urination, hematuria, urinary difficulty and urethral pain. In female patients: menstrual pain, irregular menstruation, infantile uterine fibroids and uterine prolapse.

Urethra and Vagina

Location: On the medial aspect of the heel bone, in a strip from the reflex zone of the bladder extending to the junction of the talus and navicular bones.

Indications: Urethritis, vaginitis, frequent urination, enuresis, urinary incontinence, urinary tract infections.

Rectum and Anus

Location: On the medial aspect of the ankle, in a strip between the posterior border of the tibia and the tendon of the muscle flexor hallucis longus, originating from the posterior depression to the tip of the outer malleolus.

Indications: Hemorrhoids, proctitis, rectal prolapse and constipation.

Groin

Location: On the medial aspect of the ankle, in the depression superior and anterior to the medial malleolus, on the anterior border of the tibia.

Indications: Hernia, abdominal pain and disorders of the reproductive system.

Sciatic Nerve

Location: (1) Extending from the tip of the medial malleolus, along the posterior border of the tibia to a length of approximately two palm lengths. (2) Extending from the tip of the lateral malleolus, along the anterior border of the fibula to a length of approximately two palm lengths.

Indications: Sciatica, sciatic nerve inflammation, foot numbness and leg cramps.

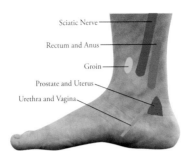

Sciatic Nerve
Rectum and Anus
Groin
Prostate and Uterus
Urethra and Vagina

FIGURE 5.9

Lower Abdomen

Location: On the posterior aspect of the lateral leg, extending upwards from the lateral malleolus to a length of proximally four finger's breadth.

Indications: Menstrual tension, irregular menstruation and abdominal pain.

Diaphragm

Location: On the dorsal aspect of the foot, crossing the cuneiform, cuboid and metatarsal bones in a strip extending from the instep.

Indications: Hiccups, nausea, vomiting, abdominal distension and abdominal pain.

Gonads (Testes and Ovaries)

Location: (1) On the plantar aspect and in the center of the heel. (2) In the triangular depression posterior and inferior to the tip of the lateral malleolus.

Indications: Dysmenorrhea, irregular menstruation, infertility, sexual dysfunction, menopausal syndrome. Reflex zones in the heel are generally named the insomnia zone, and are particularly effective in treating insomnia.

Sciatic Nerve

Location: (1) Extending from the tip of the medial malleolus, along the posterior border of the tibia to a length of approximately two palm lengths. (2) Extending from the tip of the lateral malleolus, along the anterior border of the fibula to a length of approximately two palm lengths.

Indications: Sciatica, sciatic nerve inflammation, foot numbness and leg cramps.

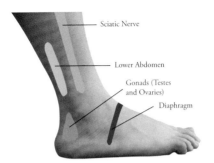

Sciatic Nerve

Lower Abdomen

Gonads (Testes and Ovaries)

Diaphragm

FIGURE 5.10

Internal Coccyx and External Coccyx

Location: Around the heel of both feet, posterior and inferior to the calcaneus bone, creating an "L" shaped strip. The medial aspect of the strip is used to treat interior coccyx conditions and the lateral aspect is used to treat external coccyx conditions.

Indications: Sciatica and sequelae of trauma to the coccyx.

Thoracic Vertebra

Location: On the medial arch of the foot, along the 1st metatarsal bone till it reaches the cuneiform junction.

Indications: Shoulder pain, thoracic bone spurs, lumbar pain, thoracic disc injury and chest pain.

Lumbar Vertebra

Location: On the medial arch of the foot, from the cuneiform bone to below the navicular bone.

Indications: Back pain, lumbar spine bone spurs, lumbar pain, lumbar disc hernia and lumbar muscle strain.

Sacrum

Location: On the medial arch of the foot, on the inside edge of the talus bone to below the calcaneus.

Indications: Sacral injuries, sacrum bone spurs and sciatica.

Hips

Location: The inferior aspects of both the medial and lateral malleoli.

Indications: Hip pain, sciatica, low back pain, weakness of the hips and numbness of the feet.

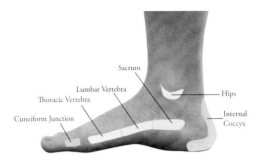

Sacrum

Lumbar Vertebra

Thoracic Vertebra

Cuneiform Junction

Hips

Internal Coccyx

FIGURE 5.11

Knee

Location: In a depression on the lateral aspect of the foot, at the junction of the 5th metatarsal bone and the anterior aspect of the calcaneus.

Indications: Knee pain, knee injuries and foot numbness.

Elbow

Location: On the lateral aspect of the foot, on the inferior part of the 5th metatarsal bone, near the metatarsal tuberosity.

Indications: Elbow pain, elbow arthritis, elbow injuries, arm and shoulder pain and numbness of the arm.

Shoulder

Location: On the lateral aspect of the 5th metatarsophalangeal joint.

Indications: Frozen shoulder, arm pain, numbness in the hand and cataracts.

Shoulder Blade

Location: On the dorsal aspect of the foot between the 4th and 5th metatarsal bones, splitting at the anterior cuboid bone to form a "Y" shape.

Indications: Frozen shoulder, shoulder pain restricted shoulder mobility.

External Coccyx

Location: Around the heel of both feet, posterior and inferior to the calcaneus bone, creating an "L" shaped strip. The medial aspect of the strip is used to treat interior coccyx conditions and the lateral aspect is used to treat external coccyx conditions.

Indications: Sciatica and sequelae of trauma to the coccyx.

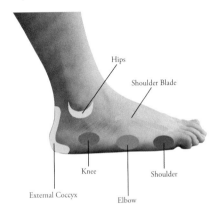

Hips

Shoulder Blade

Knee

Shoulder

External Coccyx

Elbow

FIGURE 5.12

Wrist

Location: On the dorsum of the foot, in the depression at the junction of the navicular, cuboid and articular talar bone.

Indications: Wrist pain, wrist arthritis, wrist injuries and hand numbness.

Chest (Breast)

Location: On the dorsum of the foot between the 2nd, 3rd and 4th metatarsal bones.

Indications: Chest pain, chest tightness, mastitis, breast hyperplasia, breast cancer and esophageal disease.

Ribs

Location: The medial of the two points is on the dorsum of the foot, between the 1st cuneiform bone and the scaphoid bone and is used to treat the medial ribs. The lateral of the two points is on the dorsum of the foot, between the 3rd cuneiform bone and the cuboid bone, and used to treat the lateral ribs.

Indications: Pleurisy, chest tightness, pleurisy and rib injuries.

Larynx and Trachea

Location: The lateral aspect of the 1st metatarsophalangeal joint.

Indications: Laryngitis, pharyngitis, cough, asthma, bronchitis, hoarseness and upper respiratory tract infections.

Labyrinthine

Location: On the dorsum of the foot, between the distal heads of the 4th and 5th metatarsal phalanx sutures.

Indications: Motion sickness, nausea, balance disorders, dizziness, vertigo, tinnitus, coma, hypertension, hypotension.

Maxilla and Mandibular

Location: On the dorsum of the big toe, these are two horizontal strips that cross the transverse crease of the interphalangeal joints. Use the distal strip to treat the maxilla and the proximal strip to treat the mandibular.

Indications: Tooth ache, bleeding gums, gingivitis, oral ulcers, snoring and dysgeusia.

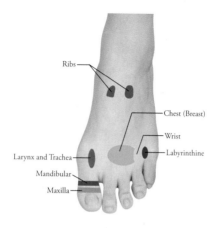

Ribs

Chest (Breast)

Wrist

Labyrinthine

Larynx and Trachea

Mandibular

Maxilla

FIGURE 5.13

Tonsils

Location: On the dorsum of the big toe, two zones either side of the tendons of the muscle extensor hallucis longus.

Indications: Tonsillitis and upper respiratory tract infection.

Chest Lymph Nodes

Location: On the dorsum of the foot, between the heads of the 1st and 2nd metatarsal bones.

Indications: Fever, inflammation, cysts and used in order to enhance the immune system's ability to fight cancer.

Cervical Lymph Nodes

Location: On the dorsum of the foot, between the distal end of each metatarsal bone, in the web at the base of each toe.

Indications: Swollen lymph nodes in the neck, goiter, hyperthyroidism and tooth ache.

Upper Body Lymph Nodes

Location: On the dorsal lateral aspect of the foot, anterior to the ankle, in the depression formed by the talus and the lateral malleolus.

Indications: Fever, inflammation, cysts and used in order to enhance the immune system's ability to fight cancer.

Lower Body Lymph Nodes

Location: On the dorsal medial aspect of the foot, anterior to the ankle, in the depression formed by the talus and the medial malleolus.

Indications: Fever, inflammation and cysts.

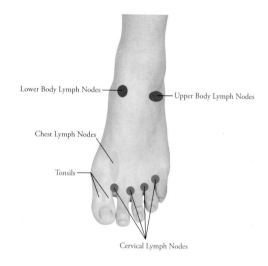

Lower Body Lymph Nodes

Upper Body Lymph Nodes

Chest Lymph Nodes

Tonsils

Cervical Lymph Nodes

FIGURE 5.14

CHAPTER 6

Wrist and Ankle Acupuncture

Wrist and ankle acupuncture is a new and simple method of shallow subcutaneous acupuncture using points on the wrist and ankle in order to treat commonly encountered conditions of the body. According to the location of the symptoms of disease, the body is divided into six vertical regions, by which selection and stimulation of six representative points on the wrist and ankle can be used for treatment. According to the regions of the body the points are selected and needled using transverse insertion to instigate sensations of soreness, numbness, swelling, heaviness and pain so as to ensure a therapeutic effect.

Differentiation and Indications

The principle of wrist and ankle acupuncture is to divide the body into six regions; the majority of conditions express specific symptoms in a distinct region of the body, analysis of the symptoms of illness can largely be attributed to one of the six longitudinal regions either on the front or back of the body. The regions are arranged along the longitudinal axis, either side of the midline. The regions are arranged as follows:

Region 1

Location: Either side of the midline, including the forehead, eyes, nose, tongue, trachea, lips, front teeth, throat, esophagus, heart, abdomen, navel, lower abdomen and perineum.

Attributed indications: Frontal headache, conditions of the eye, nasal congestion, drooling, frontal tooth ache, sore throat, bronchitis, stomach pains, palpitations, a timid nature, enuresis, dysmenorrhea and leucorrhea.

Region 2

Location: On either side of the anterior line, including the temporal region, the buccal, the posterior teeth, submandibular region, thyroid, supraclavicular fossa, the breast, lungs, liver, gallbladder on the right side of the abdomen.

Attributed indications: Frontal temporal headache, tooth ache, breast pain, chest pain, asthma, liver pain and other pain and swelling.

Region 3

Location: The outer edge of the frontal aspect of the body, including the head and face, the vertical lines anterior to the ears, the thorax and abdomen and the vertical line anterior to the lateral axilla.

Attributed indications: Few conditions manifest in the 3rd region. Superficial temporal artery disease, chest pain, abdominal pain along the axillary line.

Region 4

Location: At the junction of the anterior aspect and the posterior aspect of the body, including the side of the head to the earlobe, trapezius, chest and abdomen and the area from the armpits to the anterior superior iliac spine.

Attributed indications: Head pain, tinnitus, deafness, temporomandibular joint disorder, abdominal pain and chest conditions below the armpits.

Region 5

Location: On the outer part of the posterior aspect of the body, opposite to the anterior region 2, including the lateral temporal region, the lateral aspects of the cervical spine and the area inferior to the lateral scapula.

Attributed indications: Rear temporal head-ache, stiff neck, scapular pain and acute pain in the lumbar region.

Region 6

Location: On the lateral aspects of the posterior midline, opposite to the anterior region 1, including the back of the head, the occiput, the spine, spinous processes and transverse processes, the sacrum, coccyx and anus.

Attributed indications: Occipital headache, pain conditions, acute and chronic lumbar sprain.

In summary, the regions on the center lines are the anterior region 1, posterior region 6; the regions lateral to the central regions are the anterior region 2, posterior region 5 and the regions at the meeting of anterior and posterior parts of the body are anterior region 3, posterior region 4.

In order to establish the center point of the body, the end of the sternum and the lateral lines of the ribs indicate the costal arch, from which a horizontal line can be drawn around the body. This thereby differentiates between the upper and lower parts of the body. The regions above the horizontal line are known as the upper regions;

1 to 6, and the regions below the horizontal line are referred to as the lower regions; 1 to 6. In order to differentiate the location of symptoms based on regions, both vertical and horizontal locations can be used; for example a symptom may appear in the right hand side upper region 1, or left hand side lower region 6.

With respect to the four limbs, when both upper and lower limbs are placed in a position close to the body with the internal aspects facing the front, the internal aspects are considered the equivalent to the front of the body and the external aspects are considered equivalent to the back of the body. Therefore, the central line of the inner arm and leg are equivalent to the anterior midline of the body, similarly, the central line of the external arm and leg are equivalent to the posterior midline of the back.

Once the location of disease has been differentiated, the equivalent point on the ankle and wrist is chosen for needling. On the wrist and ankle there are six specific points, each point represents the specific region of the body, therefore, each point can be used in the treatment of diseases manifesting in the equivalent body region.

Point Location and Indications

Wrist

On the wrist there are six points circling the wrist approximately two finger's breadth proximal to the transverse crease of the wrist. The numbering of the points, Upper 1 to 6, starts from the ulna side of the palmar aspect of the wrist proceeding towards the radial side, then from the radial side of the posterior wrist towards the ulna side.

Upper 1

Location: On the side of the little finger, in a depression between the ulnar bone and the tendon of the muscle flexor carpi ulnaris.

Indications: Frontal headache, eye conditions, rhinopathy, trigeminal neuralgia, facial swelling, swelling of the front gums, pain, dizziness, sore throat, bronchitis, stomach ache, heart conditions, high blood pressure, night sweats, chills, insomnia and hysteria.

Upper 2

Location: In the center of the palmar aspect of the wrist, between the tendons of the muscles flexor carpi ulnaris and pollicis longus, at the same location of PC 6 nèi guan Inner Gate.

Indications: Anterior temporal headache, posterior tooth pain, submandibular swelling, pain, chest tightness, chest pain, delactation, asthma, angina with pain appearing in the palm (needle pointing proximally), finger numbness (needle pointing distally).

Upper 3

Location: 2 cun proximal to the transverse crease of the wrist, on the radial side of the radial artery.

Indications: High blood pressure and pain in the chest.

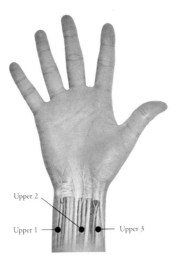

Upper 2

Upper 1

Upper 3

FIGURE 6.1

Upper 4

Location: On the posterior aspect of the forearm, on the edge of the radial bone.

Indications: Vertex headache, ear disease, temporomandibular joint dysfunction, shoulder pain, chest pain (along the axillary midline).

Upper 5

Location: In the center of the posterior aspect of the forearm, at the location on TH 5 wài guān Outer Gate.

Indications: Posterior temporal headache, upper limb sensory conditions, upper limb motor disorders, elbow joint pain, wrist and finger joint pain (needling pointing distally).

Upper 6

Location: On the edge of the ulnar bone.

Indications: Posterior headache, occipital pain and pain in the cervical and thoracic spine and paraspinal.

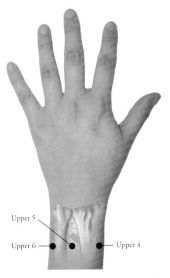

Upper 5

Upper 6 — ● ● ● — Upper 4

FIGURE 6.2

Ankle

On the ankle there are six points circling the ankle approximately three finger's breadth proximal to the medial and lateral malleolus (in an equivalent position to GB 39 xuán zhōng Suspended Bell and SP 6 sān yīn jiāo Three Leg Yin). The numbering of the points, Lower 1 to 6, starts from the medial aspect of the tendon of the Achilles and proceeds along the internal aspect of the ankle.

Lower 1

Location: On the medial edge of the tendon of the Achilles.

Indications: Upper abdominal pain, periumbilical pain, dysmenorrhea, vaginal discharge, enuresis, itching on the Yin aspect of the body and heel pain (needle pointing distally).

Lower 2

Location: In the center of medical aspect of the lower leg, on the posterior edge of the tibia.

Indications: Liver pain, pain in the lateral abdomen and allergic colitis.

Lower 3

Location: 1 cun anterior to the leading edge of the tibia.

Indications: Pain in the medial aspect of the knee.

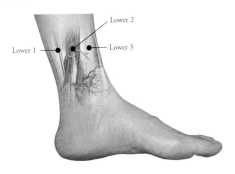

FIGURE 6.3

Lower 4

Location: At the point between the anterior aspect of the tibia and fibula.

Indications: Quadricep pain, knee pain, lower extremity sensory conditions (for example numbness and allergic reactions), lower limb movement conditions (paralysis, trembling, chorea) and toe joint pain (needle pointing distally).

Lower 5

Location: At the center of the lateral aspect of the lower leg, posterior to the fibula.

Indications: Hip pain and ankle sprain (needle pointing distally).

Lower 6

Location: Lateral to the tendon of the Achilles.

Indications: This point can be used to treat conditions in all 6 regions of the body. Acute lumbar sprain, lumbar muscle strain, sacroiliac joint pain, sciatica, gastrocnemius pain, forefoot pain (needle pointing distally).

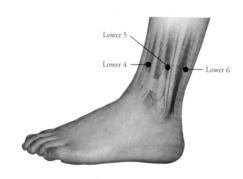

FIGURE 6.4